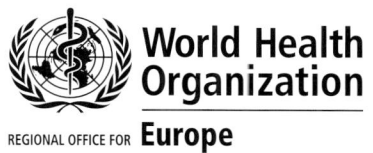

European facts and the *Global status report on road safety 2015*

Josephine Jackisch, Dinesh Sethi,
Francesco Mitis, Tomasz Szymański & Ian Arra

Abstract

In 2013, there were almost 85 000 deaths from road traffic injuries in the WHO European Region. Although the regional mortality rate is the lowest when compared to other WHO regions, with 9.3 deaths per 100 000 population, there are wide disparities in the rates of road traffic deaths between countries of the Region. This requires more systematic efforts if the global target of a 50% reduction in road crash deaths is to be achieved by 2020. Laws and practices on key risk factors such as regulating speed appropriate to road type, drink–driving, and use of seat belts, motorcycle helmets and child restraints are assessed to reduce the risk of road traffic injury. Many countries need to further strengthen their road safety legislation and enforcement in order to protect their populations, improve road user behaviour and reduce the number of crashes. While 95% of the population in the Region is covered by comprehensive laws in line with best practice for seat belts, only 47% of the population is adequately protected by laws for speed, 45% for helmet use, 33% for drink–driving and 71% for use of child restraints. Much can be gained from improving the safety of vehicles, having better road infrastructure and promoting sustainable physically active forms of mobility as alternatives to car use. Concerted policy efforts with systems approaches are needed to protect all road users in the Region.

Keywords
Accidents, Traffic - statistics and numerical data
Accidents, Traffic - trends
Wounds and injuries - epidemiology
Safety
Data collection
Europe

ISBN: 978 92 890 5126 2

Address requests about publications of the WHO Regional Office for Europe to:
    Publications
    WHO Regional Office for Europe
    UN City, Marmorvej 51
    DK-2100 Copenhagen Ø, Denmark
Alternatively, complete an online request form for documentation, health information, or for permission to quote or translate, on the Regional Office website (http://www.euro.who.int/pubrequest).

© World Health Organization 2015
All rights reserved. The Regional Office for Europe of the World Health Organization welcomes requests for permission to reproduce or translate its publications, in part or in full.

The designations employed and the presentation of the material in this publication do not imply the expression of any opinion whatsoever on the part of the World Health Organization concerning the legal status of any country, territory, city or area or of its authorities, or concerning the delimitation of its frontiers or boundaries. Dotted lines on maps represent approximate border lines for which there may not yet be full agreement.

The mention of specific companies or of certain manufacturers' products does not imply that they are endorsed or recommended by the World Health Organization in preference to others of a similar nature that are not mentioned. Errors and omissions excepted, the names of proprietary products are distinguished by initial capital letters.

All reasonable precautions have been taken by the World Health Organization to verify the information contained in this publication. However, the published material is being distributed without warranty of any kind, either express or implied. The responsibility for the interpretation and use of the material lies with the reader. In no event shall the World Health Organization be liable for damages arising from its use. The views expressed by authors, editors, or expert groups do not necessarily represent the decisions or the stated policy of the World Health Organization.

Cover photo: WHO/Faith Vorting

Contents

Acknowledgements ... iv

Abbreviations ... iv

Key facts ... 1

Background ... 1

The burden of road traffic injuries in Europe ... 1

Health systems response to road traffic injuries ... 5

National policy response to road traffic injuries and deaths ... 6

Legislation on key behavioural risk factors ... 7

    Speed ... 8

    Drink–driving ... 8

    Use of motorcycle helmets ... 10

    Use of seat belts ... 10

    Other risk factors where evidence is emerging ... 11

Other pillars of the Decade of Action for Road Safety ... 12

    Safety standards for vehicles ... 12

    Safer road infrastructure and mobility ... 13

Conclusions ... 14

References ... 14

Acknowledgements

This regional fact sheet uses data from the *Global status report on road safety 2015*. Tamitza Toroyan, Kacem Iaych and Margie Peden from WHO headquarters provided support for coordination of the project and data analysis, and valuable comments on drafts.

Country-level data were obtained with the support of the heads and staff of WHO country offices. Our thanks to national data coordinators for the work they did, questionnaire respondents and government officials who cleared the data. Francesco Mitis and Tomasz Szymanski coordinated the data collection from countries and validated the data. Joelle Auert, Leslie Zellers and Marine Perraudin helped with interpreting road safety laws.

The authors wish to thank the following for their contributions to case studies:
- Ms Anne Eriksson, Danish Road Directorate, Copenhagen, Denmark
- Ms Liza Jakobsson, Swedish Transport Agency, Solna, Sweden
- Ms Marie Skyving, Swedish Transport Agency, Solna, Sweden
- Dr Gregória Von Amann, Directorate-General of Health, Ministry of Health of Portugal, Lisbon, Portugal.

Jo Jewell and Julie Brummer from the WHO Regional Office for Europe made very helpful comments on the draft.

The authors wish to thank the following external peer reviewers for providing useful comments: Ian Roberts (London School of Hygiene & Tropical Medicine, London, United Kingdom); Elizabeth Towner (University of the West of England, Bristol, United Kingdom); Fred Wegman (SWOV Institute for Road Safety Research, Den Haag, the Netherlands); George Yannis (National Technical University of Athens, Athens, Greece) and Dave Elseroad (Global Road Safety Partnership, International Federation of Red Cross and Red Crescent Societies, Geneva, Switzerland).

The authors also thank Dr Gauden Galea, Division of Noncommunicable Diseases and Promoting Health through the Life-Course, for encouragement and support.

Generous financial support from Bloomberg Philanthropies made this analysis and publication possible.

Josephine Jackisch, Dinesh Sethi, Francesco Mitis, Tomasz Szymañski, Ian Arra
WHO Regional Office for Europe

Abbreviations

BAC	blood alcohol concentration
CIS	Commonwealth of Independent States
EFTA	European Free Trade Association
EU	European Union
GDP	gross domestic product
GNI	gross national income
HIC	high-income country
ICD-10	International Statistical Classification of Diseases and Related Health Problems, tenth revision
ISS	Injury Severity Score
LED	light-emitting diode
LMIC	low- and middle-income countries
MAIS	Maximum Abbreviated Injury Severity Score
MKD	The former Yugoslav Republic of Macedonia
SDG	Sustainable Development Goal
UN	United Nations

Key facts

> Almost 85 000 people died in the WHO European Region from road traffic injuries in 2013.

> This is a fall of 8.1% in road traffic deaths in the Region when compared to 2010, in spite of an overall increase of 7% in motor vehicles.

> Road crashes are the leading cause of death in young people aged 5–29 years.

> Almost 40% of those dying on the roads are pedestrians, cyclists and motorcyclists.

> The risk of dying from road crashes varies across the Region, with a higher risk of dying among men, children and older people, as well as populations living in low- and middle-income countries (LMIC) and countries in the eastern part of the Region.

> Mortality due to road traffic injury is almost 9 times higher in the country with the highest rate than in the country with the lowest rate.

> For every person who dies from a road crash, at least 23 have non-fatal injuries requiring hospital admissions and many more require emergency room attendances.

> Since 2010, six countries have changed laws to bring them in line with best practice on one or several of the five key risk factors.

> Preventive efforts will require considerable scaling up if the global target of a 50% reduction in road traffic deaths by 2020 is to be met.

Background

Road traffic injuries are the leading cause of premature death in young people aged 5–29 years in the WHO European Region [1]. The Decade of Action for Road Safety 2011–2020 was adopted by the United Nations General Assembly in 2010 to reduce the global toll of road traffic injuries by 2020 [2]. As a baseline for measuring progress, WHO published the *Global status report on road safety 2013: supporting a decade of action*, together with *European facts and global status report on road safety 2013* [3,4]. In September 2015, the heads of state attending the United Nations General Assembly adopted the historic Sustainable Development Goals (SDGs). These include two targets related to road safety: Goal 3.6 seeks to halve the number of global deaths and injuries from road traffic crashes by 2020, while Goal 11.2 aims to provide access to safe and sustainable transport systems [5]. In synergy with the Decade, the WHO Regional Office for Europe has proposed road safety as a priority area in *Health 2020: the European policy for health and well-being* [6]. The European Union (EU) road safety policy framework 2011–2020 also has a target of 50% reduction in fatalities by 2020 [7].

This fact sheet describes the status of road safety in 52 out of the 53 Member States of the WHO European Region, representing 95% of the Region's population.[1] It also takes stock of progress in the Region towards achieving the global target of halving the number of road traffic deaths by 2020. Experts from several sectors in each country reached consensus to complete a self-administered questionnaire under the guidance of a national data coordinator [8]. Using this method, data were collected on: (i) road traffic fatality for 2013; (ii) key policy Indicators; (iii) legislation on the established behavioural risk factors of speeding, drink–driving, and not using motorcycle helmets, seat-belts and child car restraints, as well as the emerging risk factors of mobile phone use and drug-driving; and (iv) road safety audits and mobility. Individual items of laws on the behavioural risk factors were verified using national legislative documents; this comprised a major new element of this report, with an independent expert analysis.

[1] Ukraine did not participate in this report.

Additonal information relating to vehicle standards were obtained from the database of the United Nations Economic Commission for Europe. All data were validated by national and WHO experts. A more detailed description of the methodology is provided in the *Global status report on road safety 2015* [8], where individual country profiles are also reported.

The burden of road traffic injuries in Europe

Almost 85 000 people died in road traffic injuries in the WHO European Region.

In 2013, 84 589 people died from road traffic injuries in the European Region – more than 230 every day. This constitutes a decrease of 7484 deaths or 8.1% over a three-year period from 2010 to 2013. Should the fall in the number of deaths continue at this rate, then the Region would achieve a reduction of 30% by 2020, but will fall short of the global target of a 50% reduction in fatalities. This decline nevertheless constitutes considerable success in prevention efforts *(8)*.

The European Region has the lowest road traffic mortality rate in the world, but mortality rates differ greatly between countries.

The mortality rate from road traffic injury in the European Region is 1.8 times lower than the global average (9.3 deaths per 100 000 population relative to 17.4 per 100 000 globally), and is lower than that in the other WHO regions. However, mortality rates due to road traffic injuries vary greatly across countries in the Region. Countries belonging to the Commonwealth of Independent States[2] (CIS) have a road traffic mortality rate that is three times higher than that of the European Union[3] (EU) (Fig. 1). When grouped together, road traffic mortality rates in LMIC are 1.4 times higher than in high-income countries (HICs[4]) (Fig. 2).

---

[2] CIS countries included in 2013: Armenia, Azerbaijan, Belarus, Kazakhstan, Kyrgyzstan, Republic of Moldova, Russian Federation, Tajikistan, Turkmenistan, Ukraine, Uzbekistan

[3] EU countries include the 28 Member States as of 2013: Austria, Belgium, Bulgaria, Croatia, Cyprus, Czech Republic, Denmark, Estonia, Finland, France, Germany, Greece, Hungary, Ireland, Italy, Latvia, Lithuania, Luxembourg, Malta, the Netherlands, Poland, Portugal, Romania, Slovakia, Slovenia, Spain, Sweden, the United Kingdom

[4] The World Bank Atlas method was used to categorize gross national income (GNI) into bands of: low- and middle-income = US$ 12 745 or less, and high income = US$ 12 746 or more. Where no data were available for 2013, published data for the latest year were used. From World Development Indicators database, World Bank, http://data.worldbank.org/indicator/NY.GNP.PCAP.

Mortality due to road traffic injury is 8.6 times higher in the country with the highest rate than that in the country with the lowest rate.

The lowest mortality rates are in western Europe in countries such as Sweden and the United Kingdom, whereas the highest rates are in some of the CIS countries (Fig. 3). The rate in Sweden is 8.6 times lower than the country with the highest rate. If every country achieved a similar level of road safety as Sweden, more than 59 000 lives would be saved every year. A systematic approach with concerted policy action and societal commitment is needed to reduce road traffic deaths and injuries *(8,9)*.

Fig. 1. Road traffic fatality rates per 100 000 population in countries of the Commonwealth of Independent States (CIS), WHO European Region (EUR) and European Union (EU) countries, 2013

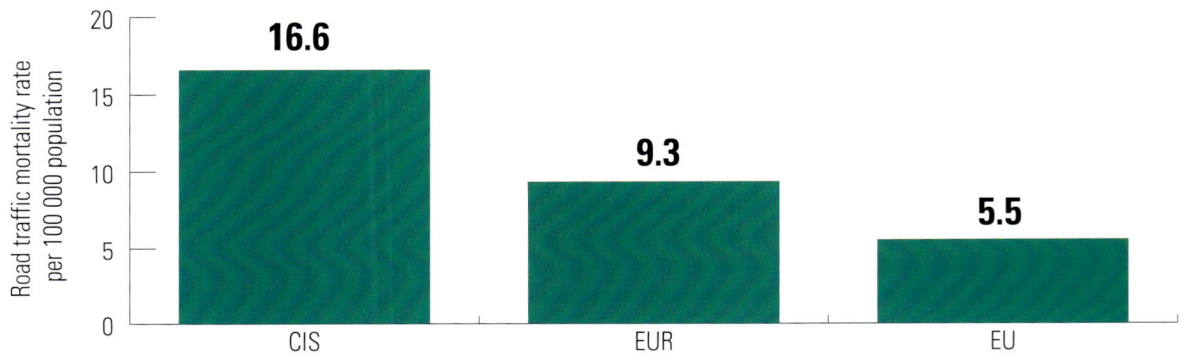

Fig. 2. Road traffic fatality rates per 100 000 population in HICs and LMIC

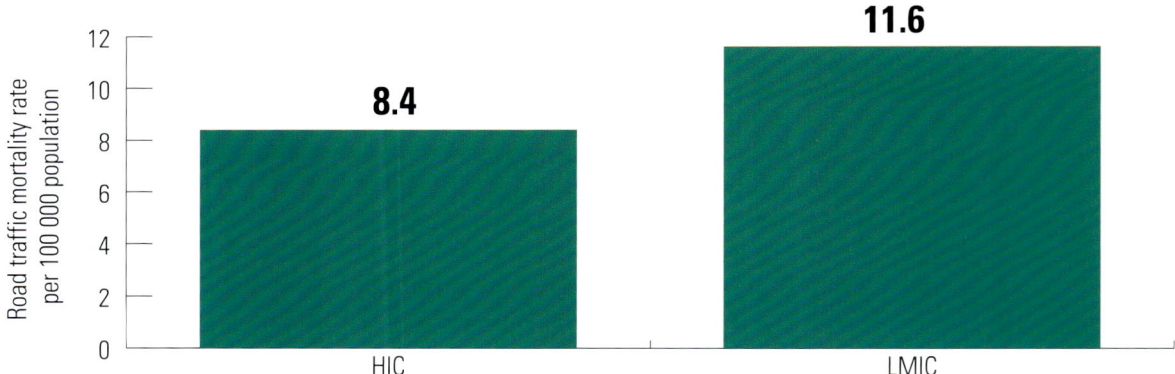

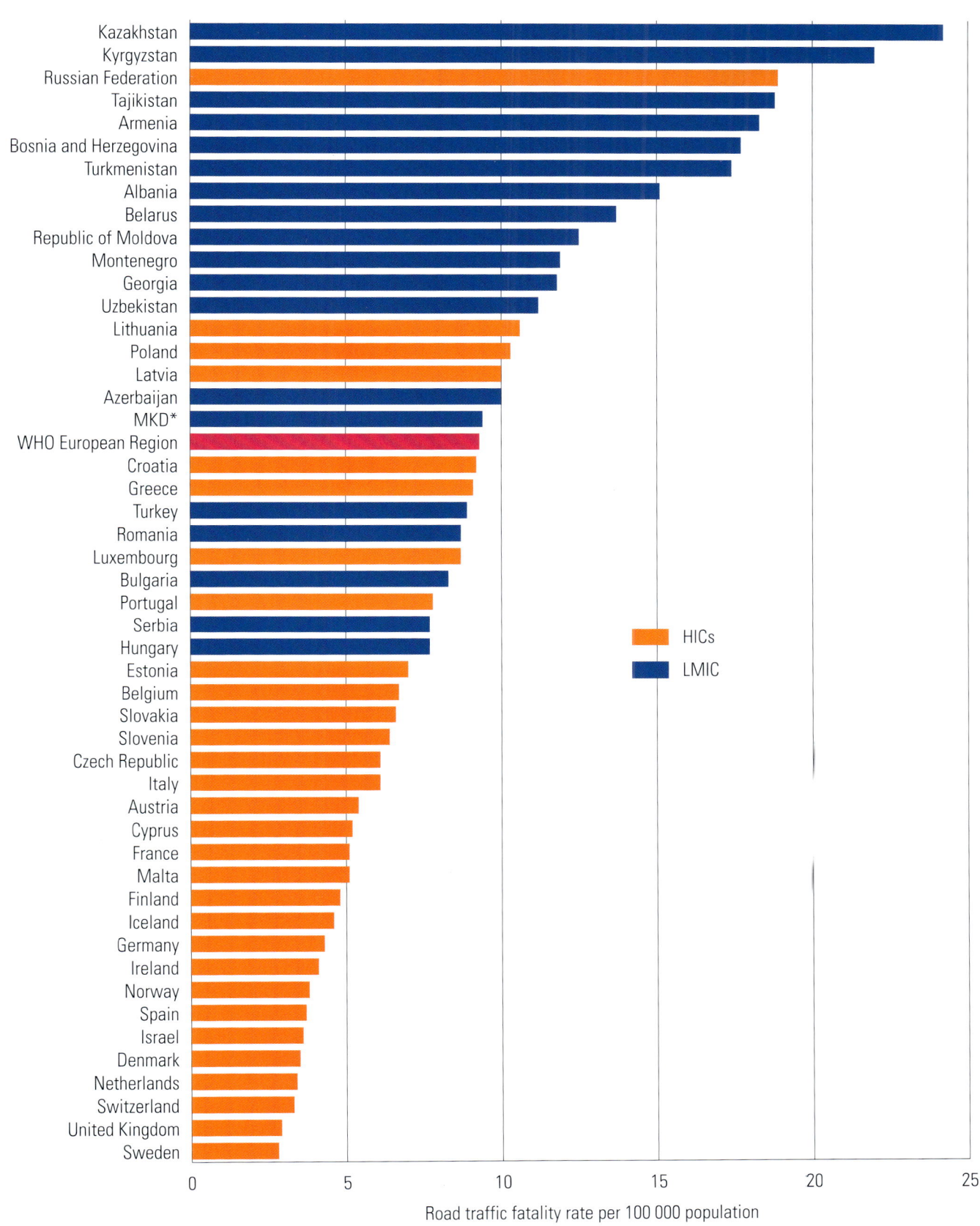

Fig. 3. Mortality rates from road traffic injuries per 100 000 population in HICs and LMIC in the WHO European Region[a,b]

[a] Data shown are for 49 out of the 52 participating countries. Those excluded have populations under 200 000. Road traffic mortality rates for the small countries in 2013: Andorra (7.6), San Marino (3.2), Monaco (did not record any fatalities in this period).
[b] Modelled mortality rates; for details of the modelling process please see the *Global status report on road safety 2015 (8)*.
* MKD is the International Organization for Standardization abbreviation for The former Yugoslav Republic of Macedonia.

Forty countries reported fewer road traffic deaths in 2013 than in 2010.

Forty countries have made progress in reducing the number of road crash deaths (Fig. 4).[5] The European Region achieved an overall 8.1% reduction in deaths between 2010 and 2013, despite an increase of 7% in the number of registered vehicles in the same period. Motorization has been higher at 29% in countries belonging to the CIS. Nevertheless, some countries such as the Russian Federation have managed to limit the increase in the number of deaths to less than 2% despite a 17% increase in vehicles through sustained policy interventions.

Almost 4 out of 10 deaths are in pedestrians, cyclists and motorcyclists.

In total, 39% of deaths are among pedestrians, cyclists and motorcyclists, who are not well protected from the impact of a crash (Fig. 5). Compared with the European Region and the EU, the proportion of pedestrian deaths is highest in the CIS countries; the proportions of cyclist and motorcyclist deaths are highest in the EU.

Road traffic fatalities are just the tip of the iceberg.

Data on deaths do not convey the full story of the magnitude of harm caused by road crashes. There is little systematically collected information on the severity of injuries, resulting disabilities and devastating impact on people's lives, the burden to health-care systems and costs to society as a whole. In 2013, countries in the Region reported a total of 1.6 million non-fatal injuries. This suggests that for every reported death, there are on average 23 injured people. Previous studies from EU countries allow estimates of the non-fatal injury burden across the EU. Between 2008 and 2010, for every person who died from road traffic injury, 18 people were admitted to hospital and another 92 people were treated as hospital outpatients – amounting to 110 non-fatal road traffic injuries for each fatality (10). This suggests that the reported figures

---

[5] These data represent countries that have seen more than a 2% change in their number of deaths since 2010, and excludes countries with populations under 200 000. Countries with populations of less than one million are more likely to be affected by statistical uncertainty and annual variations may appear large due to the small numbers.

Fig. 4. Number of countries with increased and decreased number of deaths in 2013 compared to 2010 in the European Region, CIS and EU countries[5]

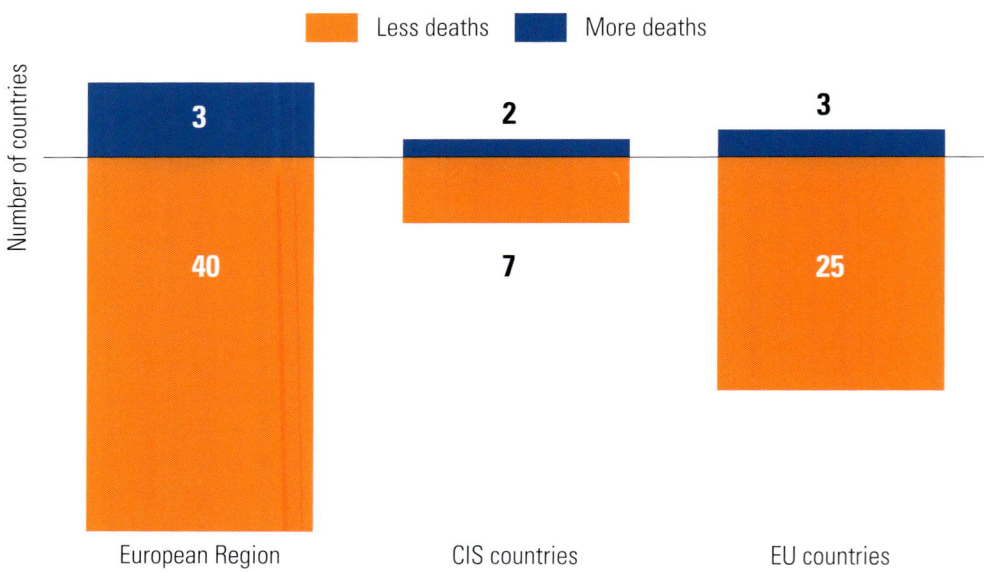

Fig. 5. Distribution of deaths by type of road user in the European Region, CIS and EU

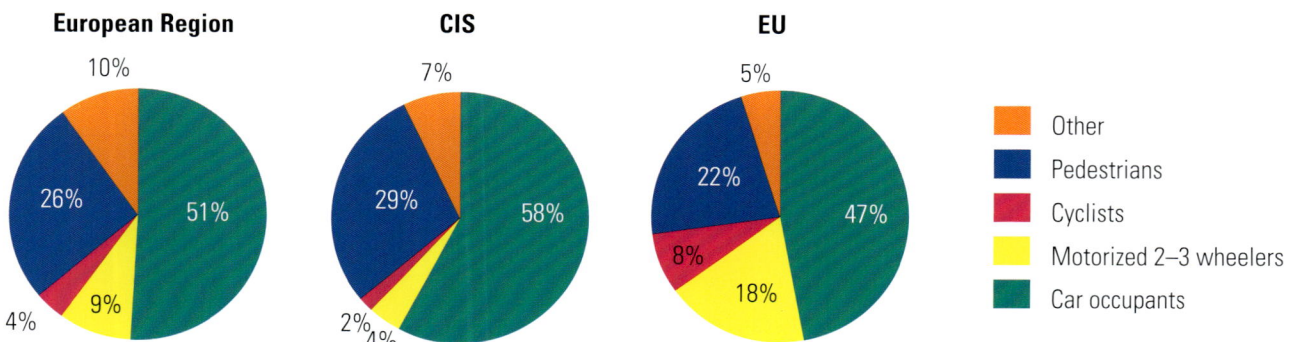

of non-fatal road traffic injuries might be an underestimate of the size of the problem.

Road traffic injury mortality rates are highest in young males.

Mortality rates due to road traffic injuries also vary by age and gender. Rates are highest in young people aged 15–29 years, older people aged 70 years or more, and are three times higher in males than females (Fig. 6).

Many road traffic injuries have drastic consequences for the individuals involved and their families.

Road traffic injuries can have a devastating impact on people's lives. The humanitarian consequences are also vast. Information on the far-reaching consequences of road crashes on people's lives is scarce. For example, only 13 countries[6] provide estimates of the proportion of road traffic crashes resulting in a permanent disability; these range from 0.5% to 11.5%, with a median of 4% (latest data available between 2008 and 2013). These data are likely to underestimate the scale of the problem and better information is needed.

---

[6] The 13 countries reporting the proportion of road traffic crashes resulting in a permanent disability are: Austria, Azerbaijan, Croatia, Finland, Greece, Italy, Kazakhstan, Luxembourg, the Netherlands, San Marino, Slovakia, Sweden, the former Yugoslav Republic of Macedonia.

The economic burden to society warrants increased action across all sectors in countries.

Thirty-one countries have conducted studies to calculate the economic costs of road crashes as a proportion of their gross domestic product (GDP). These estimates reported societal costs, which ranged from 0.6% to 5.8% of the GDP, with a median of 1.4% of the GDP. More estimates are needed using a standardized methodology.

Health systems' response to road traffic injuries

Post-crash response can save lives – many countries need to improve their emergency trauma services.

Efficient and high-quality emergency services can improve outcomes and survival after a crash. Some of the disparity in mortality rates in the Region may be attributable to better-quality post-crash response and emergency care in some countries, resulting in improved survival, as has been reported from HICs (11). Rapid access to such care is critical. Forty-two countries have a universal nationwide emergency telephone number. Thirty-two countries reported that their ambulance services take 75% or more of those seriously injured on the roads to hospital. This was true for 70% of the HICs and 47% of the LMIC.

Health systems capacity in emergency trauma care needs to be strengthened.

Efficient emergency trauma care requires specially trained staff. Emergency medicine is recognized as a specialty for medical doctors in 41 countries – this remains unchanged since 2010. Forty countries now recognize emergency medicine as a postgraduate training programme for nurses, four more than in 2010.

Injury surveillance systems need to be improved and emergency room-based data collected.

Data on road traffic injuries is essential for monitoring progress towards national targets, and evaluating prevention programmes and the quality of post-crash care. All 52 responding countries monitor road deaths through police databases but five countries use definitions that are shorter than the international standard of assessing death within 30 days of a crash.[7] Further, 47 countries also have good-quality vital registration data for national estimates of mortality using the International Statistical Classification of Diseases and

---

[7] The 30-day defintion of a road crash death applies to a person who dies within 30 days of a crash on a public road involving a vehicle with an engine, the death being the result of the crash. Such data are collated by the authority responsible for road crash data and are usually notified by the police.

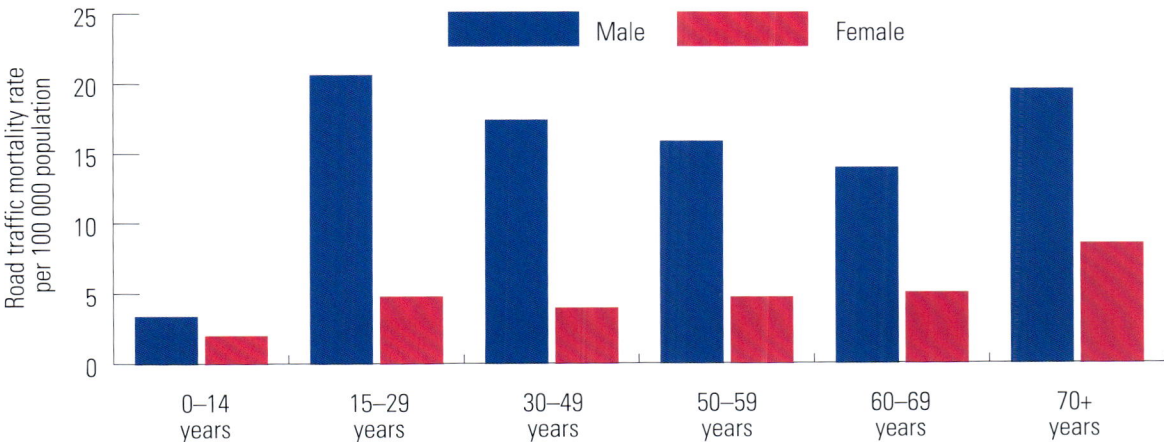

Fig. 6. Mortality rates in the WHO European Region from road traffic injuries per 100 000 population by age and gender, 2012

Source: Global health estimates (1)

Related Health Problems, tenth revision (ICD-10) *(8)* or an equivalent system of registration *(12)*. Only 10 countries report data linkage between police and vital registration data to improve official mortality statistics.[8]

Surveillance of non-fatal injuries and assessment of injury severity remains a challenge. Many countries depend on police reports of those who are admitted to hospitals, while others also include less severe injuries treated in emergency departments. Different sources of data, coding practices and definitions create a challenge for monitoring non-fatal injuries. In health-care facilities, 31 countries use the ICD-10 for classifying the severity of injuries, seven use the Abbreviated Injury Score *(13)* (or its derivatives, the Maximum Abbreviated Injury Severity Score (MAIS) and Injury Severity Score [ISS]), others use national systems of severity grading and six countries do not classify the severity of injuries at all. Many countries in the EU collect data using the MAIS to monitor severe road traffic injuries *(14)*. Having a reliable injury surveillance system that measures injury severity is essential for monitoring targets to reduce severe road traffic injuries. Twenty countries report that they do not have a national emergency room-based surveillance system.

National policy response to road traffic injuries and deaths

Most countries in Europe have developed national strategies to improve road safety.

National road safety strategies have been developed in 49 out of the 52 countries that took part in the survey, suggesting that road safety is high on their policy agenda. The presence of agencies tasked with improving road safety was reported in 49 countries, three more than in 2010. National road safety strategies or plans require the combined actions of many sectors and such agencies are best placed to coordinate such actions, as proposed by the Decade of Action for Road Safety *(2)*.

National road safety targets are a valuable tool for ensuring the implementation of national road safety strategies. Forty-four countries have set measurable targets to reduce deaths and 23 to also reduce the number of the seriously injured. Many countries also have specific targets to improve the risk factors of speed, drink–driving, and use of seat-belts, child restraints and helmets (Fig. 7).

[8] Azerbaijan, Estonia, Finland, Israel, Luxembourg, the Netherlands, Portugal, Romania, the Russian Federation and Spain report this.

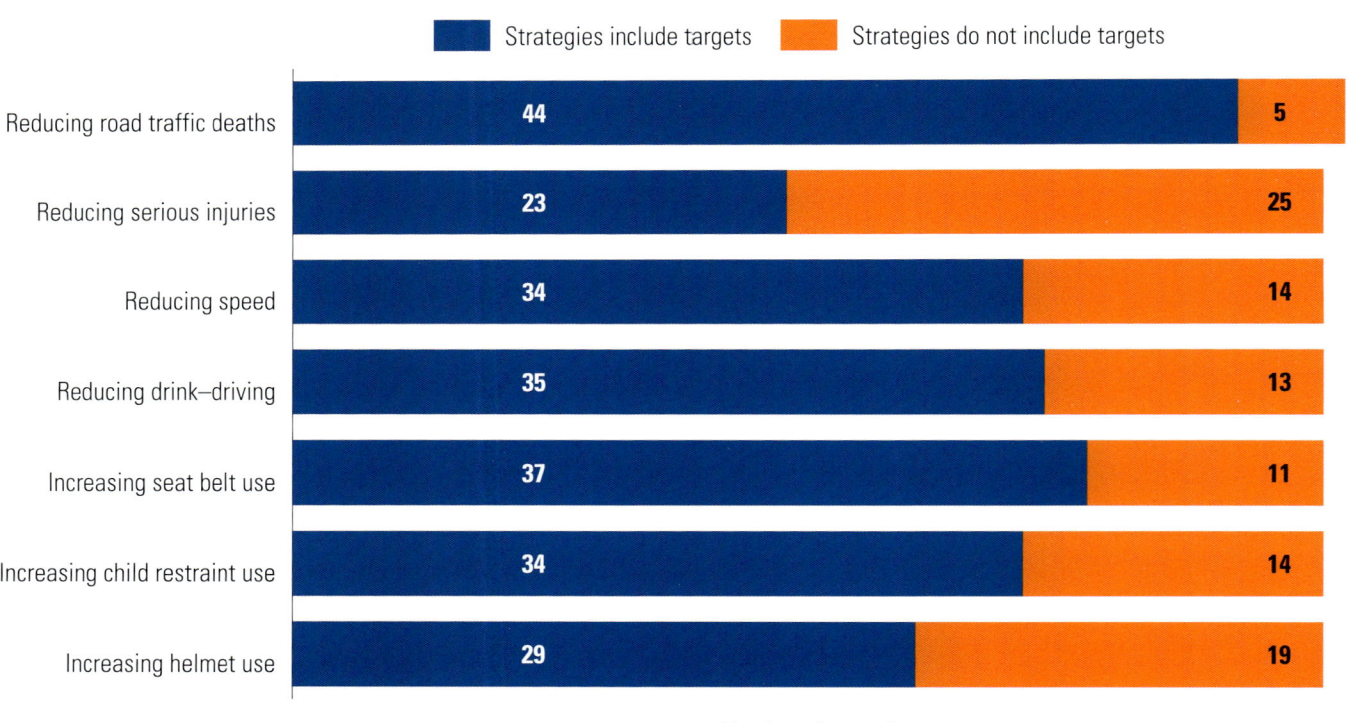

Fig. 7. Number of countries with national road safety strategies with specific targets

- Strategies include targets
- Strategies do not include targets

Category	Include targets	Do not include targets
Reducing road traffic deaths	44	5
Reducing serious injuries	23	25
Reducing speed	34	14
Reducing drink–driving	35	13
Increasing seat belt use	37	11
Increasing child restraint use	34	14
Increasing helmet use	29	19

Number of countries

Legislation on key behavioural risk factors

Adopting and enforcing comprehensive laws is an effective way of improving road user behaviour to enhance safety on the roads. There is a strong evidence base showing that laws addressing the key risk factors of speeding, drink–driving, non-use of motorcycle helmets, seat-belts and child restraints can reduce road traffic deaths and injuries (8,9,15,16). In order to be effective, such laws need to be in line with best practice and properly enforced. The working definitions of comprehensive laws on these risk factors are described in Box 1. Evidence is also emerging on the potential risks of mobile phone use while driving, and driving under the influence of drugs.

Enforcement of laws is essential to changing risk behaviours and needs to be improved.

Enforcement of the existing laws varies widely in the Region. Twenty countries reported a high level of enforcement for seat-belt legislation but only five countries reported this for speed (a score of 8 or more on a scale of 1 to 10). Clearly, much more needs to be done to enhance enforcement in many countries (Fig. 8). Laws enforced by traffic police should result in the administration of penalities commensurate with the severity of the offence. These range from driving license demerit or penalty points, to administrative fines, licence withdrawal, vehicle impoundment and even imprisonment. Risk behaviour is best modified if enforcement is coordinated with social marketing campaigns (9).

> **Box 1. Criteria used to define comprehensive legislation for key behavioural risk factors**
>
> **Speed:** a national speed limit law with a maximum urban speed limit of 50 km/h and the power of local authorities to reduce speed limits to ensure safe speeds locally
>
> **Drink–driving:** a national drink–driving law based on a blood alcohol concentration (BAC) of ≤0.05 g/dl for the general population and a BAC of ≤0.02 g/dl for novice drivers
>
> **Motorcycle helmets:** a national law on motorcycle helmet use that applies to all drivers and passengers, on all roads and all engine types, and requires the helmet to be fastened and which makes reference to a particular helmet standard
>
> **Seat belts:** a national law on seat-belt use that applies to all private car occupants on front and rear seats
>
> **Child restraints:** a national law on the use of child restraints based on age, height or weight of a child, and the existence of a law that applies age or height restrictions to children sitting in the front seat
>
> These criteria constitute international best practice as defined in the *Global status report on road safety 2015 (8)*.

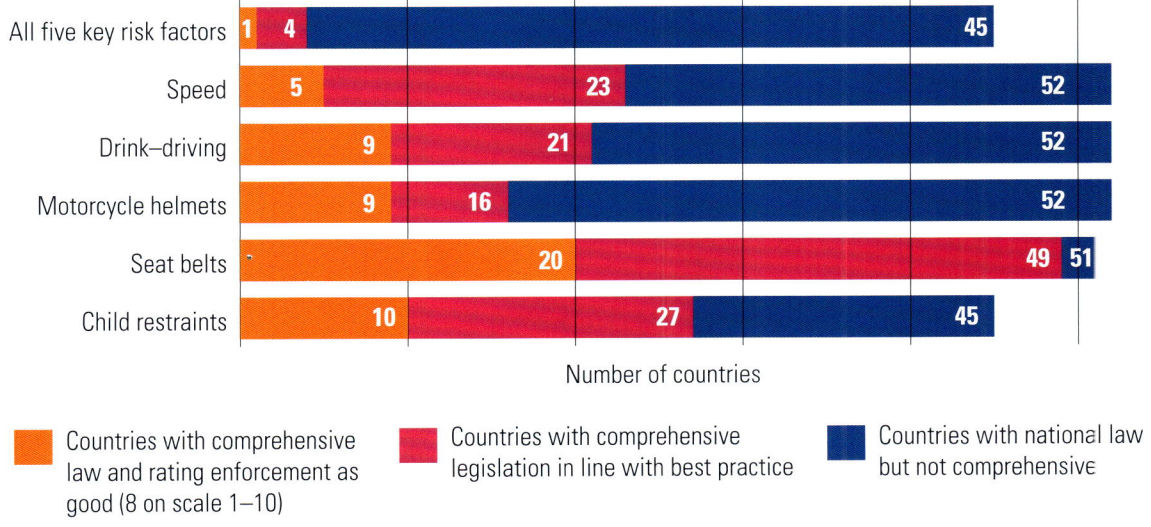

Fig. 8. Number of countries with legislation for the five risk factors and whether these are comprehensive and well enforced

Speed

Reducing urban speed limits is key to protecting pedestrians and cyclists.

High speed increases the likelihood of a crash, as well as serious injury and death in the event of a crash. In urban areas where motorized traffic meets pedestrians, cyclists and motorcycle riders, speed limits need to take account of the safety of all road users *(8,14,15)*. Forty-four per cent (23 of 52) of countries have comprehensive speed regulations, which consist of a national urban speed limit ≤50 km/h and giving local authorities the permission to lower those limits. This covers 47% of the population in the European Region, as shown in the map in Fig. 9. However, enforcement needs to be improved (Fig. 8). While 38 countries out of 52 (73%) have urban speed limits of 50 km/h or less, 14 countries still have an urban speed limit exceeding 50 km/h.

Speed limits should be reduced to 30 km/h in areas where vulnerable road users and cars mix, for example, around schools and residential areas. It is therefore important to give local authorities the power to lower speed limits for such conditions. However, almost half of the countries in the Region (48%) do not allow local authorities to lower national speed limits. Fifteen countries could reach the status of comprehensive speed legislation by granting local authorities this authority.

Enforcement of existing speed limits needs to be improved.

People who violate speed regulations face fines (in 49 countries), licence withdrawal (34 countries) or demerit points (28 countries). Only five countries report that enforcement of their respective speed laws is effective (≥8 on a scale from 1 to 10); three are HICs and two are LMIC. Social marketing campaigns can help to support enforcement.

Fig. 9. National speed laws on urban roads, by country

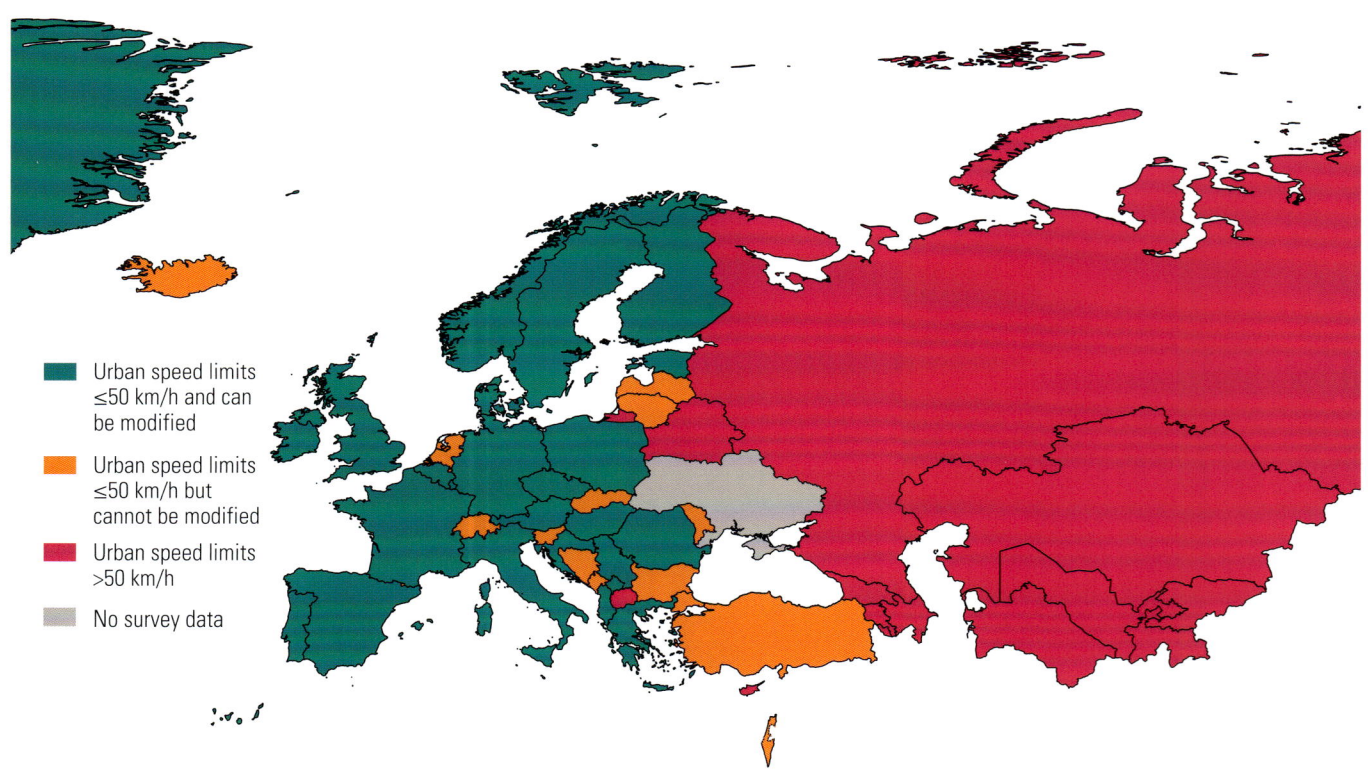

Drink–driving

All countries in the European Region have national laws to regulate drink–driving but in only 22 countries are these in line with best practice.

Current best practice requires national legislation with a drink–driving law, based on a maximum BAC of 0.05 g/dl for the general population and ≤0.02 g/dl for novice drivers. Since 2011, three countries (Ireland, Switzerland and Portugal) have changed their drink–driving laws to be in line with these criteria for best practice.

Eleven countries do not have a lower limit for novice drivers, six countries do not base their law on objective measures such as BAC, and four countries allow a maximum BAC of 0.08 g/dl (Fig. 10).[9]

---
[9] Countries with a maximum legal BAC of 0.08 g/dl for drivers in the general population are: Armenia, Malta, Romania, United Kingdom

Fig. 10. Drink–driving legislation by country

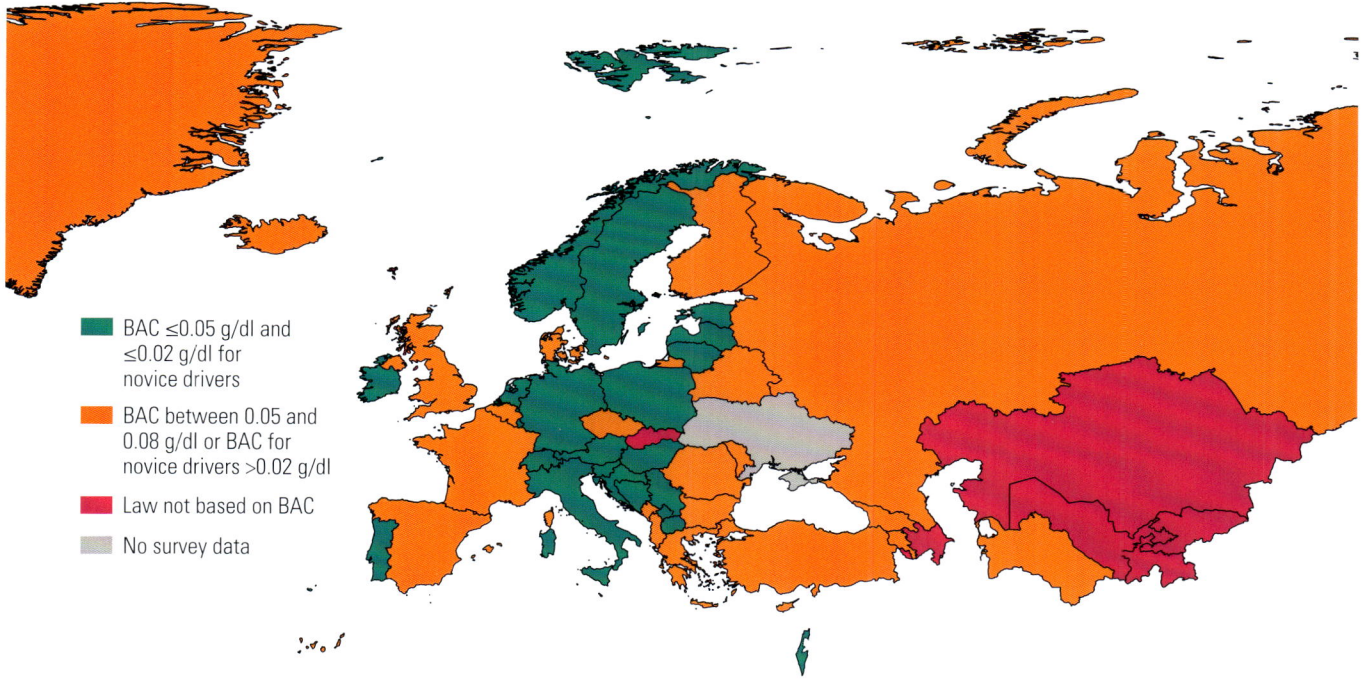

- BAC ≤0.05 g/dl and ≤0.02 g/dl for novice drivers
- BAC between 0.05 and 0.08 g/dl or BAC for novice drivers >0.02 g/dl
- Law not based on BAC
- No survey data

In order to be effective, the enforcement of drink–driving laws needs to be supported by BAC testing as well as by strict penalties and social marketing campaigns. In the WHO European Region, 94% of countries use all year-round random breath testing to enforce the laws, and 77% of countries use breath testing in specific locations (e.g. pubs) or at specific times.

A median of 14% of road traffic deaths are attributable to drinking and driving.

National estimates of the proportion of road traffic deaths that are attributable to alcohol use are collected in 46 countries and range from less than 1% to 31%, with a median of 14%. Only 39 countries give police the authority to test BAC in drivers involved in fatal injury crashes, though this may not be routinely practised. Better and more complete data on BAC testing are needed in countries to estimate the potential of preventing drink–driving and reduce alcohol-related harm. Box 2 provides an example of a systematic approach to tackling the problem of drink–driving.

Box 2. Case study Sweden: a comprehensive systems approach to drink–driving

Sweden has adopted the Safe System approach (8) to road safety. As part of this progress to safer roads, Sweden has been the front runner in the fight against drink–driving. A number of interrelated policy and programmatic interventions have contributed to Sweden's success.

› The Swedish Government has made drink–driving one of its highest priorities with a cohesive strategy that includes preventive work for the whole society (17).

› Permissible BAC levels were reduced to 0.02 g/dl for all drivers.

› The "Vision Zero" target (15) has empowered both individuals and the community to strive for safer roads.

› There is a high frequency and visibility of law enforcement by the police in tackling drink–driving, as demonstrated by the large number of breath tests per population.

› Education on the negative effects of alcohol and drugs is mandatory when applying for a driver's license.

› There is widespread public awareness of the dangers of drink–driving and high public acceptance of the countermeasures being implemented to address the problem; this has been achieved through social marketing campaigns.

› Alcohol interlocks are used widely in commercial transport, government vehicles and school buses, and as a complementary component of rehabilitation programmes.

› Rehabilitation programmes aim to provide medical treatment for problem drinking rather than punishing the offender. The SMADIT programme (Samverkan Mot Alkohol och Droger i Trafiken [collaboration against alcohol and drugs in traffic]) takes a systematic approach towards this.

Use of motorcycle helmets

Progress has been made in protecting motorcyclists but few countries have laws that meet best practice and are well enforced.

The proportion of motorcycle deaths in the WHO European Region decreased from 12% to 9% of all traffic deaths between 2010 and 2013. The number of registered motorized two- and three-wheelers has hardly changed. All countries in the WHO European Region have laws in place that make helmet use compulsory for motorized two-wheelers. However, only 16 countries have laws that meet all the criteria of best practice. In 27 countries, safety standards for helmets have not been adopted (Fig. 11). In two countries, laws on helmet-wearing do not apply to all engine types, while in 21 countries, the law does not stipulate that helmets need to be properly fastened.

Overall, 32 countries (61%) reported that the enforcement of helmet laws by police is effective. Only nine countries have comprehensive legislation that is well enforced (Fig. 8). Twenty-seven countries collect data on the number of motorcycle riders who wear helmets. Seventeen of those who collect data found helmet-wearing rates at 90% or above; eight countries have lower helmet-wearing rates. In general, helmet-wearing rates were lower in passengers than in drivers.

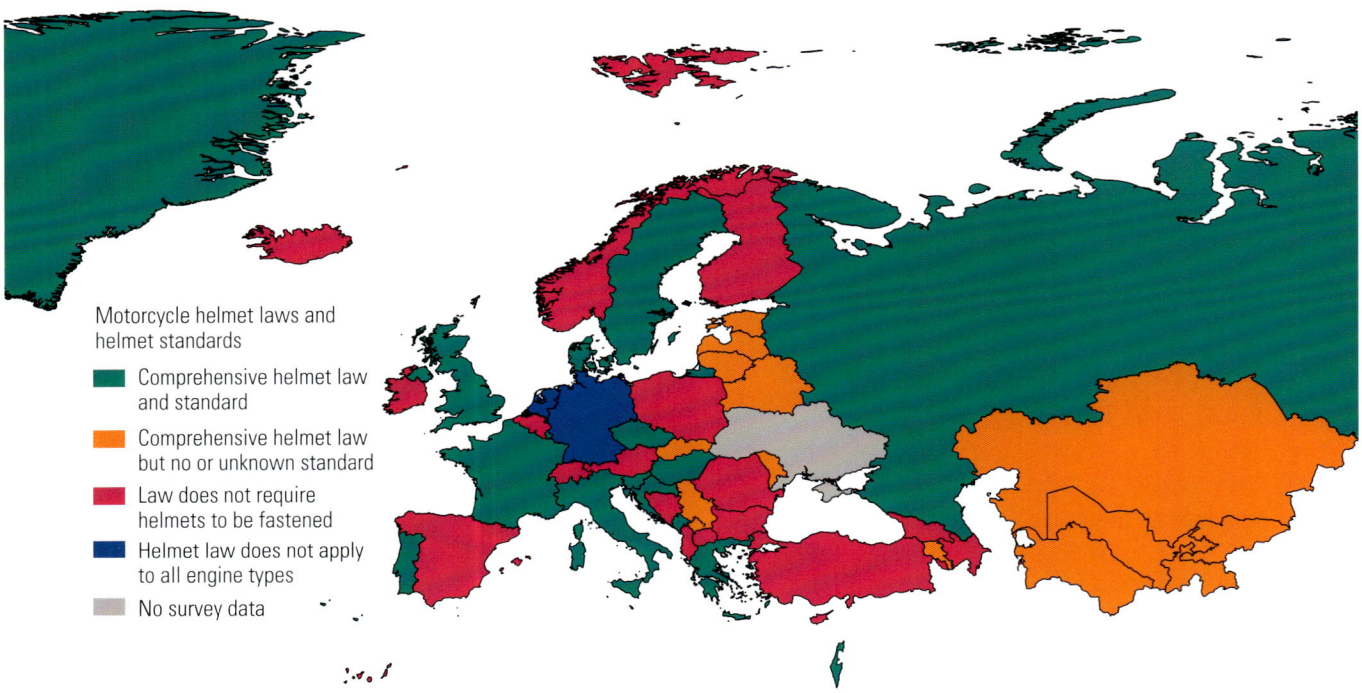

Fig. 11. Legislation on use of motorcycle helmets by country

Use of seat belts

Forty-nine countries have comprehensive laws on seat belt use, covering 94.5% of the Region's population.

Comprehensive laws on seat-belt use are those that cover both front and rear seat occupants in private cars. Some countries apply exceptions; while a few may be justified, others put road users at unnecessary risk. Turkmenistan recently brought their law in line with good practice.

National data on rates of wearing seat belts are suboptimal in many countries, suggesting that enforcement needs to be improved.

Only 20 countries (42%) rate their enforcement as effective, suggesting that it needs to be improved. Collecting data on the proportion of people wearing seat belts is essential to evaluating the effectiveness of enforcement and seat-belt wearing campaigns. Such data are not available in 16 countries on front seat-belt use and 19 countries on rear seat-belt use (Table 1). For the 36 countries that measure seat-belt wearing among front seat occupants, the median reported usage was 86%. The median proportion of rear seat-belt use was 65% in the 32 countries that collect this data. Box 3 provides an example of how enhanced enforcement and social marketing campaigns were used to improve seat-belt wearing.

Use of child restraints in cars needs to be increased.

Forty-five countries (87%) have laws on the use of child restraints in cars based on age, height or weight; however, only 29 countries also restrict children from sitting in the front seat (Fig. 12). Since 2011, Montenegro and Turkey have brought their child-restraint laws

Fig. 12. Legislation on car child restraint by country

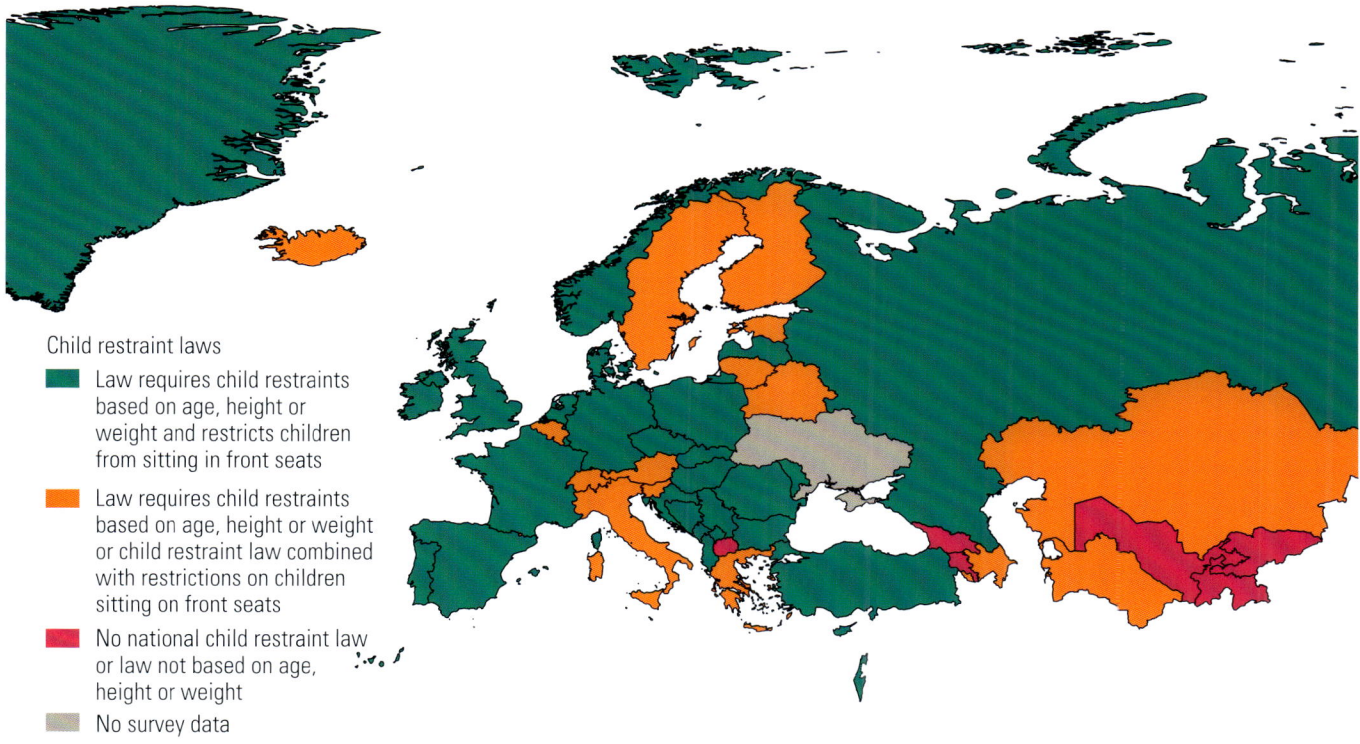

Child restraint laws
- ■ Law requires child restraints based on age, height or weight and restricts children from sitting in front seats
- ■ Law requires child restraints based on age, height or weight or child restraint law combined with restrictions on children sitting on front seats
- ■ No national child restraint law or law not based on age, height or weight
- ■ No survey data

Table 1. Number of countries with legislation, enforcement and data on seat-belt use

Laws, enforcement and data availability on seat-belt use	HICs N=33	LMICs N=19	Total N=52	%
Seat-belt use				
Countries in which all car occupants are required to use seat belts in front and rear seats in line with comprehensive legislation	31	18	49	94%
Countries with comprehensive law and enforcement ≥8 (scale of 1 to 10)[a]	14	6	20	42%[a]
Countries with no data on seat-belt usage, front seats	6	10	16	31%
Countries with no data on seat-belt usage, rear seats	6	13	19	37%

[a] Calculated for the 48 countries where a consensus on the effectiveness of law enforcement was reached.

in line with best practice. Box 4 provides an example of a systematic approach to encouraging child-restraint use.

Other risk factors where evidence is emerging

In some areas, such as mobile phone use and drug-driving, better evidence is emerging regarding the harm caused by these and the effectiveness of interventions (8).

Drug-driving laws need to be more concrete.

There is growing recognition of the problem of driving under the influence of drugs, especially if used in combination with alcohol (8). All countries except for one have national laws against drug-driving. While in most countries these laws generally apply to legal and illegal drugs that impair driving, only nine countries specify what these are. Enforcement of these laws remains a challenge, as best practice in testing for drugs and hence enforcement is only just emerging. Only 22 countries routinely test drivers involved in fatal crashes for drugs.

Mobile phone use poses a risk by distracting drivers.

Being distracted while driving significantly increases the risk of crashes. Mobile phone use is a major cause of distracted driving. Evidence is accumulating on the risk that mobile phone use poses to road safety.

Box 3. Intersectoral action to improve the use of seat belts and child restraints in two Russian regions

An intersectoral road safety project was implemented in two Russian regions, Lipetsk and Ivanovo, between 2010 and 2014. The project was supported by Bloomberg Philanthropies and implemented by a consortium of international, national and regional partners, including WHO, the Ministry of Interior and Ministry of Health. One of its aims was to increase seat-belt use by vehicle occupants in both the front and rear seats, and to increase child-restraint use.

Increased seat-belt and child-restraint use was achieved through social marketing campaigns to modify risk behaviours, enhanced enforcement to reinforce the messages of safe behaviours, building local police and administrative capacities to enable this, evaluation consisting of 3–6-monthly roadside measurements to assess adoption of safety behaviours, and engaging the media to disseminate the messages. Courses were also run in first aid for drivers and the police. Over a period of 4 years, the project resulted in an increase in the use of seat belts and child restraints by 25–41 and 33–69 percentage points, respectively. This project demonstrated how investing in collaboration between the transport, justice/interior and health sectors at both the national and regional levels was essential for achieving the project objectives. The social marketing tools, measurement tools, capacity-building materials and information on organizational approaches are stored on an accessible website to facilitate their use in other regions in the Russian Federation *(18)*.

Box 4. Case study Portugal: safety of babies, children and youth

Safe transport of babies and children is a political priority in Portugal for both the Ministry of Health and the Ministry of Internal Affairs. Triggered by the Decade of Action for Road Safety, on 11 May 2011, a joint project was launched by the two ministries with the aim of ensuring safe transportation of newborn babies starting from hospital maternity wards, and maintaining this through childhood. The National Road Safety Strategy for 2008–2015 reinforces this in its strategic and operational objectives, and the National Programme of Injury Prevention developed a project called "Safety of Babies, Children and Youth", aiming to reduce child mortality and serious injury by increasing the use of child-restraint systems.

Measures included legislation mandating that all vehicles, including buses and coaches that transport children, are equipped with child-restraint systems. Another intervention targeted paediatric hospitals and paediatricians, who had to train parents of newborn children about the importance of using child safety restraints and provide them with child safety training, including on the correct use of child restraints. Currently, there are projects being implemented in 47 hospitals and health centres, involving 6000 health professionals who have trained over 60 000 parents. In the near future, the project will start working with grandparents. Portugal has been one of the leaders in reducing child mortality due to traffic collisions, with an annual average reduction of 15% in road mortality among children in 2009. This success was a result of the adoption of multiple and collaborative strategies and interventions, which require local partnerships between the Portuguese Government, the private sector, foundations (such as the MAPFRE Foundation) and nongovernmental organizations (such as the Portuguese Association for Child Safety Promotion) *(19,20)*. This collaboration has led to successful local implementation.

Fifty countries (96%) prohibit hand-held phone use while driving. Evidence suggests that hands-free phones have no significant advantage over hand-held phones in terms of reducing the risk of crashes *(8)*. Only four countries prohibit the use of hands-free phones while driving. No country routinely collects data on mobile phone use while driving.

Other pillars of the Decade of Action for Road Safety

Safety standards for vehicles

Safety standards for vehicles in an important pillar of the Decade of Action for Road Safety *(2)*. The number of vehicles on the roads is increasing in the Region, in particular, in the eastern part. There is growing concern about whether these vehicles meet international vehicle safety standards *(8)*. Vehicle safety standards guide vehicle makers in manufacturing vehicles that reduce the likelihood of crashes, protect car occupants from harm in the event of a crash and minimize damage to other road users, such as pedestrians. Seven of the United Nations (UN) safety standards for new cars[10] set by the UN World Forum for Harmonization of Vehicle Regulations were prioritized to assess safety in this report. All EU and European Free Trade Association (EFTA) countries plus Turkey and the Russian Federation apply the seven key safety standards for frontal impact, side impact, electronic stability control, pedestrian protection, seat belts, seat-belt anchorages, child restraints; but many other countries do not. Where such vehicle standards are absent or not enforced, automobile companies are able to sell models without these safety features, putting populations at greater risk.

---

[10] These include standards for frontal impact, side impact, electronic stability control, pedestrian protection, seat belts, seat-belt anchorages, child restraints *(8)*.

Safer road infrastructure and mobility

More countries should conduct formal road assessments for safety.

Safer road infrastructure is another important goal of the Decade of Action for Road Safety *(2)*. In the Region, 49 countries (94%) require safety reviews for the design and planning of new road infrastructure. Fifty-one countries (98%) inspect existing infrastructure for safety on a regular basis, mainly through maintenance safety inspections (79%), and 34 countries (65%) conduct formal road assessments for safety. Many countries and municipalities also perform crash black spot analyses and safety audits to make existing roads safer.

Sustainable transport is a win–win strategy by making roads safer and the population healthier.

The health and development benefits of linkages between sustainable transport and road safety have been emphasized in the SDGs 2016–2030 *(5)*. Physically active forms of transport such as walking and cycling have health benefits as they counteract the likelihood of developing obesity and noncommunicable diseases *(21)*. This is also true of public transport, which requires more walking than private car use. Dependence on motor vehicle transport causes environmental damage due to air pollution, noise pollution and climate change. These in turn have health-damaging effects such as respiratory illness, cardiovascular disease, cancer, as well as the dangers of extreme weather events and the impact on mental well-being *(15)*.

Thirty per cent of all road traffic deaths in the Region occur among pedestrians and cyclists, and much more should be done to protect these vulnerable road users, particularly when considering the population health benefits of physically active mobility. Thirty-three countries in the Region have national policies that encourage walking and cycling, and a further 10 countries have these at subnational level. Physically active transport is encouraged by the WHO European Physical Activity Strategy 2016–2025 *(21)*.

These important efforts need to go hand in hand with increasing the protection of vulnerable road users and ensuring that walking and cycling become safer (Box 5). Thirty-two countries have national policies to protect pedestrians and cyclists by physically separating them from motorized traffic. In 12 countries, such policies exist at the subnational level, while eight countries have no policy in place for separating vulnerable road users from high-speed traffic. Besides promoting walking and cycling, countries should also promote public transport as alternatives to car travel. Thirty-five countries have national and another nine subnational policies to support investment in public transport. This is three countries more than in 2010.

Box 5. Copenhagen: a city with sustainable and safe cycling

Every day, 63% of Copenhagen's residents use a bicycle for their daily commute to work. Safe transport planning has been at the heart of this success. This was through two traffic safety plans by the City of Copenhagen for the periods 2000–2012 and 2007–2012 *(22)*. A comprehensive set of road safety policies and interventions were introduced to help all road users make the safest choices in traffic. These include the following:

❯ improved infrastructure for cyclists, with raised cycle tracks, bridges and parking;

❯ lowering speed limits to 40 km/h in all residential areas and on stretches of road where vulnerable road users cross the road, such as all school gates and all shopping streets;

❯ accident analysis and identification of dangerous locations or "black spot analysis";

❯ reducing the number of potential conflicts between road users by improving junctions and intersections: marking of cycle lanes at intersections, and other measures to make drivers more aware of cyclists when turning, and signalized intersections with light-emitting diode (LED) lights to alert lorry drivers about oncoming cyclists;

❯ using garbage trucks with low cabins so that drivers have a better view of cyclists before turning.

❯ a Safe Routes to School programme that focuses on making schoolchildren more competent as cyclists and pedestrians;

❯ higher helmet usage rates for cyclists due to campaigns and smarter designs;

❯ better driver education and campaigns, and more effective and targeted police control;

❯ incorporating road safety audits and planning in all urban development projects.

These plans have resulted in a 35% fall in the number of deaths and serious injuries when comparing the average for the period 2003–2005 to that for 2012. When broken down, this shows a 21% decrease in deaths for cyclists, 51% for scooter and moped drivers, 27% for pedestrians and 58% for cars. Furthermore, the large number of cyclists has contributed to greater safety, as car drivers have become more aware of cyclists.

Conclusions

Road traffic injuries are a big health challenge for countries in the WHO European Region. Road traffic crashes resulted in 84 590 deaths in 2013, an estimated 1.6 million hospital admissions and numerous more emergency room attendances. There has been an 8.1% reduction in deaths (7484 in number) in the Region since 2010.

There are large inequalities in the rates of road traffic injuries in the Region, with the largest number of deaths in the eastern part of the Region. The Region also has some countries with the lowest road traffic mortality in the world, such as Sweden, the United Kingdom, Switzerland and the Netherlands. These reductions have been the result of sustained efforts over a period of 50 years and by implementing the Safe System approach to road safety *(8,15)*. Such approaches and the lessons learnt from the many success stories need to be applied elsewhere in Europe. Reaching the ambitious SDG target of a 50% reduction in road crash deaths by 2020 will be a challenge unless there is greater political will to confront the problem, with systematic and coordinated action across multiple sectors. In addressing these, physically active mobility should be encouraged to counteract obesity and the threat of noncommunicable diseases. This fact sheet presents the Region's achievements since the baseline assessment for 2010, highlights weaknesses and risks, and proposes actions to encourage Member States of the European Region to achieve greater safety on their roads. The following actions are proposed:

› National road safety strategies with targets that are monitored are useful tools to achieve road safety. These strategies need to involve many sectors. Whereas national road safety strategies exist in the majority of countries, more countries need to have strategies that include targets to reduce mortality and severe injuries due to crashes.

› Better injury surveillance systems and data related to these are needed to monitor progress towards these targets.

› Changing road user behaviour is an essential part of achieving safety on the roads, as much of the risk of crashing is due to risky behaviour. The enactment of laws that meet best practice is one way of modifying road user behaviour. Whereas the majority of countries have laws (87%), these laws need to be strengthened in many countries to bring them in line with best practice.

› Laws are effective in changing risky behaviour only if well enforced. The majority of countries report that there needs to be better enforcement of existing laws. Optimal enforcement practices need to be better understood. Social marketing campaigns would help better enforcement and acceptance of laws by the public.

› Pedestrians, cyclists and motorcyclists make up 39% of the deaths on the roads in the Region. Making walking and cycling safer, and providing public transport will encourage people to use these physically active and sustainable forms of transport. This would provide additional health and environmental benefits.

› The adoption of international vehicle safety standards is essential to making cars safer on the roads. Only 36 countries in the Region meet the priority safety standards assessed. More countries need to implement these standards to prevent harm to all road users from crashes.

› More countries need to conduct formal road safety assessments.

› Greater investment is needed in emergency and health systems capacity to improve the post-crash quality of care in many countries.

References

1. WHO Global health estimates 2014 summary tables: Deaths by cause, age and sex, by WHO region, 2000–2012 (http://www.who.int/healthinfo/global_burden_disease/en/, accessed 01 October 2015).

2. The Global Plan for a Decade of Action for Road Safety 2011–2020. New York: United Nations Road Safety Collaboration; 2010 (http://www.who.int/roadsafety/decade_of_action/plan/en/, accessed 03 November 2015).

3. Global status report on road safety 2013: supporting a decade of action. Geneva: World Health Organization; 2013 (http://www.who.int/violence_injury_prevention/road_safety_status/2013/en/, accessed 03 November 2015).

4. European facts and global status report on road safety 2013. Copenhagen: WHO Regional Office for Europe; 2013 (http://www.euro.who.int/en/publications/abstracts/european-facts-and-global-status-report-on-road-safety-2013, accessed 1 October 2015).

5. Transforming our world: the 2030 Agenda for Sustainable Development. New York: United Nations General Assembly: 2015 [A/70/L.1] (https://sustainabledevelopment.un.org/topics, accessed 01 October 2015)

6. Health 2020: a European policy framework supporting action across government and society for health and well-being. Copenhagen: WHO Regional Office for Europe; 2012 [EUR/RC62/9] (http://www.euro.who. int/__data/assets/pdf_file/0009/169803/RC62wd09-Eng.pdf, accessed 01 October 2015).

7. Road safety study for the interim evaluation of Policy Orientations on

Road Safety 2011–2020. Brussels: European Commission; 2015 (http://ec.europa.eu/transport/road_safety/pdf/study_final_report_february_2015_final.pdf, accessed 01 October 2015).

8. Global status report on road safety 2015. Geneva: World Health Organization; 2015 (http://www.who.int/violence_injury_prevention/road_safety_status/2015/en/, accessed 03 November 2015).

9. Peden M, Scurfield R, Sleet D, Mohan D, Hyder AA, Jarawan E, et al., editors. World report on road traffic injury prevention. Geneva: World Health Organization; 2004.

10. Injuries in the European Union: summary of injury statistics for the years 2008–2010. Amsterdam: EuroSafe; 2013 (http://ec.europa.eu/health/data_collection/docs/idb_report_2013_en.pdf, accessed 01 October 2015).

11. Guidelines for essential trauma care. Geneva: World Health Organization; 2004 (http://www.who.int/violence_injury_prevention/publications/services/guidelines_traumacare/en, accessed 01 October 2015).

12. ICD-10: International Statistical Classification of Diseases and Related Health Problems, tenth revision, second edition. Geneva: World Health Organization; 2004 (http://apps.who.int/iris/handle/10665/42980, accessed 01 October 2015).

13. Abreviated Injury Scale – 2005. update 2008 [webpage]. Chicago: Association for the Advancement of Automative Medicine; 2015 (http://www.aaam.org/about-ais.html, accessed 01 October 2015).

14. High-level group on road safety consultation on the development of the injuries strategy: next steps in the development of the injuries strategy. Brussels: European Commission; 2012 (http://ec.europa.eu/transport/road_safety/pdf/injury_next_steps.pdf, accessed 03 November 2015).

15. Racioppi F, Eriksson L, Tingvall C, Villaveces A. Preventing road traffic injury: a public health perspective for Europe. Copenhagen: WHO Regional Office for Europe; 2004 (http://www.euro.who.int/__data/assets/pdf_file/0003/87564/E82659.pdf, accessed 03 November 2015).

16. Global status report on road safety: time for action. Geneva: World Health Organization; 2009 (http://whqlibdoc.who.int/publications/2009/9789241563840_eng.pdf, accessed 01 October 2015).

17. A cohesive strategy for alcohol, narcotic drugs, doping and tobacco (ANDT) policy. Ministry of Health and Social Affairs, Sweden; 2011 [S.2011.02] (http://www.government.se/information-material/2011/05/a-cohesive-strategy-for-alcohol-narcotic-drugs-doping-and-tobacco-andt-policy/ accessed 01 October 2015).

18. Kondratiev V, Shikin V, Grishin V, Orlov S, Klyavin V, et al. Intersectoral action to improve road safety in two regions of the Russian Federation. Public Health Panorama. 2015;1:192–7.

19. MAPFRE Foundation. Children's road safety [website] (https://babyseat.fundacionmapfre.org/children/, accessed 01 October 2015).

20. 20. APSI: the Portuguese Association for Child Safety Promotion [website] (http://www.apsi.org.pt/index.php/pt/, accessed 01 October 2015).

21. Physical activity strategy for the WHO European Region 2016–2025. Copenhagen: WHO Regional Office for Europe; 2015 [EUR/RC65/9] http://www.euro.who.int/__data/assets/pdf_file/0010/282961/65wd09e_PhysicalActivityStrategy_150474.pdf?ua=1, accessed 03 November 2015).

22. Copenhagen 2013–2020: traffic safety plan. Copenhagen: The city of Copenhagen; 2013 (http://kk.sites.itera.dk/apps/kk_pub2/pdf/1154_iGUpXeTKoQ.pdf, accessed 01 October 2015).